MINIATURE GOLF SCORECARD

Course Location:

Date:

Player	1	2	3	4	5				
Par									

Player	10	11	12	13	14	15	16	17	18	Total
Par										

Notes:

MINIATURE GOLF SCORECARD

Course Location:

Date:

Player	1	2	3	4	5	6	7	8	9
Par									

Player	10	11	12	13	14	15	16	17	18	Total
Par										

Notes:

MINIATURE GOLF SCORECARD

Course Location:

Date:

Player	1	2	3	4	5	6	7	8	9
Par									

Player	10	11	12	13	14	15	16	17	18	Total
Par										

Notes:

MINIATURE GOLF SCORECARD

Course/Location:
Date:

Player	1	2	3	4	5	6	7	8	9
Par									

Player	10	11	12	13	14	15	16	17	18	Total
Par										

Notes:

MINIATURE GOLF SCORECARD

Course Location:

Date:

Player	1	2	3	4	5	6	7	8	9
Par									

Player	10	11	12	13	14	15	16	17	18	Total
Par										

Notes:

MINIATURE GOLF SCORECARD

Course/Location:

Date:

Player	1	2	3	4	5	6	7	8	9
Par									

Player	10	11	12	13	14	15	16	17	18	Total
Par										

Notes:

MINIATURE GOLF SCORECARD

Course Location:

Date:

Player	1	2	3	4	5	6	7	8	9
Par									

Player	10	11	12	13	14	15	16	17	18	Total
Par										

Notes:

MINIATURE GOLF SCORECARD

Course/Location:

Date:

Player	1	2	3	4	5	6	7	8	9
Par									

Player	10	11	12	13	14	15	16	17	18	Total
Par										

Notes:

MINIATURE GOLF SCORECARD

Course Location:

Date:

Player	1	2	3	4	5	6	7	8	9
Par									

Player	10	11	12	13	14	15	16	17	18	Total
Par										

Notes:

MINIATURE GOLF SCORECARD

Course/Location:

Date:

Player	1	2	3	4	5	6	7	8	9
Par									

Player	10	11	12	13	14	15	16	17	18	Total
Par										

Notes:

MINIATURE GOLF SCORECARD

Course Location:

Date:

Player	1	2	3	4	5	6	7	8	9
Par									

Player	10	11	12	13	14	15	16	17	18	Total
Par										

Notes:

MINIATURE GOLF SCORECARD

Course/Location:

Date:

Player	1	2	3	4	5	6	7	8	9
Par									

Player	10	11	12	13	14	15	16	17	18	Total
Par										

Notes:

MINIATURE GOLF SCORECARD

Course Location:

Date:

Player	1	2	3	4	5	6	7	8	9
Par									

Player	10	11	12	13	14	15	16	17	18	Total
Par										

Notes:

MINIATURE GOLF SCORECARD

Course Location:

Date:

Player	1	2	3	4	5	6	7	8	9
Par									

Player	10	11	12	13	14	15	16	17	18	Total
Par										

Notes:

Course Location:

Date:

Player	1	2	3	4	5	6	7	8	9
Par									

Player	10	11	12	13	14	15	16	17	18	Total
Par										

Notes:

| Course/Location: |
| Date: |

Player	1	2	3	4	5	6	7	8	9
Par									

Player	10	11	12	13	14	15	16	17	18	Total
Par										

Notes:

MINIATURE GOLF SCORECARD

Course Location:

Date:

Player	1	2	3	4	5	6	7	8	9
Par									

Player	10	11	12	13	14	15	16	17	18	Total
Par										

Notes:

MINIATURE GOLF SCORECARD

Course/Location:

Date:

Player	1	2	3	4	5	6	7	8	9
Par									

Player	10	11	12	13	14	15	16	17	18	Total
Par										

Notes:

MINIATURE GOLF SCORECARD

Course Location:

Date:

Player	1	2	3	4	5	6	7	8	9
Par									

Player	10	11	12	13	14	15	16	17	18	Total
Par										

Notes:

MINIATURE GOLF SCORECARD

Course Location:

Date:

Player	1	2	3	4	5	6	7	8	9
Par									

Player	10	11	12	13	14	15	16	17	18	Total
Par										

Notes:

MINIATURE GOLF SCORECARD

Course Location:

Date:

Player	1	2	3	4	5	6	7	8	9
Par									

Player	10	11	12	13	14	15	16	17	18	Total
Par										

Notes:

MINIATURE GOLF SCORECARD

Course/Location:
Date:

Player	1	2	3	4	5	6	7	8	9
Par									

Player	10	11	12	13	14	15	16	17	18	Total
Par										

Notes:

MINIATURE GOLF SCORECARD

Course Location:

Date:

Player	1	2	3	4	5	6	7	8	9
Par									

Player	10	11	12	13	14	15	16	17	18	Total
Par										

Notes:

MINIATURE GOLF SCORECARD

Course Location:

Date:

Player	1	2	3	4	5	6	7	8	9
Par									

Player	10	11	12	13	14	15	16	17	18	Total
Par										

Notes:

Course Location:

Date:

Player	1	2	3	4	5	6	7	8	9
Par									

Player	10	11	12	13	14	15	16	17	18	Total
Par										

Notes:

MINIATURE GOLF SCORECARD

Course Location:

Date:

Player	1	2	3	4	5	6	7	8	9
Par									

Player	10	11	12	13	14	15	16	17	18	Total
Par										

Notes:

MINIATURE GOLF SCORECARD

Course Location:

Date:

Player	1	2	3	4	5	6	7	8	9
Par									

Player	10	11	12	13	14	15	16	17	18	Total
Par										

Notes:

MINIATURE GOLF SCORECARD

Course/Location:

Date:

Player	1	2	3	4	5	6	7	8	9
Par									

Player	10	11	12	13	14	15	16	17	18	Total
Par										

Notes:

MINIATURE GOLF SCORECARD

Course Location:

Date:

Player	1	2	3	4	5	6	7	8	9
Par									

Player	10	11	12	13	14	15	16	17	18	Total
Par										

Notes:

MINIATURE GOLF SCORECARD

<table>
<tr><td>Course Location:</td></tr>
<tr><td>Date:</td></tr>
</table>

Player	1	2	3	4	5	6	7	8	9
Par									

Player	10	11	12	13	14	15	16	17	18	Total
Par										

Notes:

MINIATURE GOLF SCORECARD

Course Location:

Date:

Player	1	2	3	4	5	6	7	8	9
Par									

Player	10	11	12	13	14	15	16	17	18	Total
Par										

Notes:

MINIATURE GOLF SCORECARD

Course/Location:

Date:

Player	1	2	3	4	5	6	7	8	9
Par									

Player	10	11	12	13	14	15	16	17	18	Total
Par										

Notes:

MINIATURE GOLF SCORECARD

Course Location:

Date:

Player	1	2	3	4	5	6	7	8	9
Par									

Player	10	11	12	13	14	15	16	17	18	Total
Par										

Notes:

MINIATURE GOLF SCORECARD

Course/Location:

Date:

Player	1	2	3	4	5	6	7	8	9
Par									

Player	10	11	12	13	14	15	16	17	18	Total
Par										

Notes:

MINIATURE GOLF SCORECARD

<table>
<tr><td>Course Location:</td></tr>
<tr><td>Date:</td></tr>
</table>

Player	1	2	3	4	5	6	7	8	9
Par									

Player	10	11	12	13	14	15	16	17	18	Total
Par										

Notes:

MINIATURE GOLF SCORECARD

Course/Location:

Date:

Player	1	2	3	4	5	6	7	8	9
Par									

Player	10	11	12	13	14	15	16	17	18	Total
Par										

Notes:

MINIATURE GOLF SCORECARD

Course Location:

Date:

Player	1	2	3	4	5	6	7	8	9
Par									

Player	10	11	12	13	14	15	16	17	18	Total
Par										

Notes:

MINIATURE GOLF SCORECARD

Course Location:

Date:

Player	1	2	3	4	5	6	7	8	9
Par									

Player	10	11	12	13	14	15	16	17	18	Total
Par										

Notes:

MINIATURE GOLF SCORECARD

Course Location:

Date:

Player	1	2	3	4	5	6	7	8	9
Par									

Player	10	11	12	13	14	15	16	17	18	Total
Par										

Notes:

MINIATURE GOLF SCORECARD

Course/Location:

Date:

Player	1	2	3	4	5	6	7	8	9
Par									

Player	10	11	12	13	14	15	16	17	18	Total
Par										

Notes:

MINIATURE GOLF SCORECARD

Course Location:

Date:

Player	1	2	3	4	5	6	7	8	9
Par									

Player	10	11	12	13	14	15	16	17	18	Total
Par										

Notes:

MINIATURE GOLF SCORECARD

Course/Location:
Date:

Player	1	2	3	4	5	6	7	8	9
Par									

Player	10	11	12	13	14	15	16	17	18	Total
Par										

Notes:

MINIATURE GOLF SCORECARD

Course Location:

Date:

Player	1	2	3	4	5	6	7	8	9
Par									

Player	10	11	12	13	14	15	16	17	18	Total
Par										

Notes:

MINIATURE GOLF SCORECARD

Course Location:

Date:

Player	1	2	3	4	5	6	7	8	9
Par									

Player	10	11	12	13	14	15	16	17	18	Total
Par										

Notes:

MINIATURE GOLF SCORECARD

Course Location:

Date:

Player	1	2	3	4	5	6	7	8	9
Par									

Player	10	11	12	13	14	15	16	17	18	Total
Par										

Notes:

MINIATURE GOLF SCORECARD

Course/Location:

Date:

Player	1	2	3	4	5	6	7	8	9
Par									

Player	10	11	12	13	14	15	16	17	18	Total
Par										

Notes:

MINIATURE GOLF SCORECARD

Course Location:

Date:

Player	1	2	3	4	5	6	7	8	9
Par									

Player	10	11	12	13	14	15	16	17	18	Total
Par										

Notes:

MINIATURE GOLF SCORECARD

Course Location:

Date:

Player	1	2	3	4	5	6	7	8	9
Par									

Player	10	11	12	13	14	15	16	17	18	Total
Par										

Notes:

MINIATURE GOLF SCORECARD

Course Location:

Date:

Player	1	2	3	4	5	6	7	8	9
Par									

Player	10	11	12	13	14	15	16	17	18	Total
Par										

Notes:

MINIATURE GOLF SCORECARD

Course Location:

Date:

Player	1	2	3	4	5	6	7	8	9
Par									

Player	10	11	12	13	14	15	16	17	18	Total
Par										

Notes:

MINIATURE GOLF SCORECARD

Course Location:

Date:

Player	1	2	3	4	5	6	7	8	9
Par									

Player	10	11	12	13	14	15	16	17	18	Total
Par										

Notes:

MINIATURE GOLF SCORECARD

Course/Location:
Date:

Player	1	2	3	4	5	6	7	8	9
Par									

Player	10	11	12	13	14	15	16	17	18	Total
Par										

Notes:

MINIATURE GOLF SCORECARD

Course Location:

Date:

Player	1	2	3	4	5	6	7	8	9
Par									

Player	10	11	12	13	14	15	16	17	18	Total
Par										

Notes:

MINIATURE GOLF SCORECARD

Course/Location:

Date:

Player	1	2	3	4	5	6	7	8	9
Par									

Player	10	11	12	13	14	15	16	17	18	Total
Par										

Notes:

MINIATURE GOLF SCORECARD

Course Location:

Date:

Player	1	2	3	4	5	6	7	8	9
Par									

Player	10	11	12	13	14	15	16	17	18	Total
Par										

Notes:

MINIATURE GOLF SCORECARD

Course Location:

Date:

Player	1	2	3	4	5	6	7	8	9
Par									

Player	10	11	12	13	14	15	16	17	18	Total
Par										

Notes:

MINIATURE GOLF SCORECARD

Course Location:

Date:

Player	1	2	3	4	5	6	7	8	9
Par									

Player	10	11	12	13	14	15	16	17	18	Total
Par										

Notes:

Course/Location:

Date:

Player	1	2	3	4	5	6	7	8	9
Par									

Player	10	11	12	13	14	15	16	17	18	Total
Par										

Notes:

MINIATURE GOLF SCORECARD

Course Location:

Date:

Player	1	2	3	4	5	6	7	8	9
Par									

Player	10	11	12	13	14	15	16	17	18	Total
Par										

Notes:

MINIATURE GOLF SCORECARD

Course/Location:

Date:

Player	1	2	3	4	5	6	7	8	9
Par									

Player	10	11	12	13	14	15	16	17	18	Total
Par										

Notes:

MINIATURE GOLF SCORECARD

Course Location:

Date:

Player	1	2	3	4	5	6	7	8	9
Par									

Player	10	11	12	13	14	15	16	17	18	Total
Par										

Notes:

MINIATURE GOLF SCORECARD

Course/Location:

Date:

Player	1	2	3	4	5	6	7	8	9
Par									

Player	10	11	12	13	14	15	16	17	18	Total
Par										

Notes:

MINIATURE GOLF SCORECARD

Course Location:

Date:

Player	1	2	3	4	5	6	7	8	9
Par									

Player	10	11	12	13	14	15	16	17	18	Total
Par										

Notes:

MINIATURE GOLF SCORECARD

| Course Location: |
| Date: |

Player	1	2	3	4	5	6	7	8	9
Par									

Player	10	11	12	13	14	15	16	17	18	Total
Par										

Notes:

MINIATURE GOLF SCORECARD

Course Location:

Date:

Player	1	2	3	4	5	6	7	8	9
Par									

Player	10	11	12	13	14	15	16	17	18	Total
Par										

Notes:

MINIATURE GOLF SCORECARD

Course/Location:

Date:

Player	1	2	3	4	5	6	7	8	9
Par									

Player	10	11	12	13	14	15	16	17	18	Total
Par										

Notes:

MINIATURE GOLF SCORECARD

Course Location:

Date:

Player	1	2	3	4	5	6	7	8	9
Par									

Player	10	11	12	13	14	15	16	17	18	Total
Par										

Notes:

MINIATURE GOLF SCORECARD

Course Location:

Date:

Player	1	2	3	4	5	6	7	8	9
Par									

Player	10	11	12	13	14	15	16	17	18	Total
Par										

Notes:

MINIATURE GOLF SCORECARD

Course Location:

Date:

Player	1	2	3	4	5	6	7	8	9
Par									

Player	10	11	12	13	14	15	16	17	18	Total
Par										

Notes:

MINIATURE GOLF SCORECARD

| Course/Location: |
| Date: |

Player	1	2	3	4	5	6	7	8	9
Par									

Player	10	11	12	13	14	15	16	17	18	Total
Par										

Notes:

MINIATURE GOLF SCORECARD

Course Location:

Date:

Player	1	2	3	4	5	6	7	8	9
Par									

Player	10	11	12	13	14	15	16	17	18	Total
Par										

Notes:

MINIATURE GOLF SCORECARD

Course Location:

Date:

Player	1	2	3	4	5	6	7	8	9
Par									

Player	10	11	12	13	14	15	16	17	18	Total
Par										

Notes:

MINIATURE GOLF SCORECARD

Course Location:

Date:

Player	1	2	3	4	5	6	7	8	9
Par									

Player	10	11	12	13	14	15	16	17	18	Total
Par										

Notes:

MINIATURE GOLF SCORECARD

Course Location:

Date:

Player	1	2	3	4	5	6	7	8	9
Par									

Player	10	11	12	13	14	15	16	17	18	Total
Par										

Notes:

MINIATURE GOLF SCORECARD

Course Location:

Date:

Player	1	2	3	4	5	6	7	8	9
Par									

Player	10	11	12	13	14	15	16	17	18	Total
Par										

Notes:

MINIATURE GOLF SCORECARD

Course/Location:

Date:

Player	1	2	3	4	5	6	7	8	9
Par									

Player	10	11	12	13	14	15	16	17	18	Total
Par										

Notes:

MINIATURE GOLF SCORECARD

Course Location:

Date:

Player	1	2	3	4	5	6	7	8	9
Par									

Player	10	11	12	13	14	15	16	17	18	Total
Par										

Notes:

MINIATURE GOLF SCORECARD

Course/Location:

Date:

Player	1	2	3	4	5	6	7	8	9
Par									

Player	10	11	12	13	14	15	16	17	18	Total
Par										

Notes:

MINIATURE GOLF SCORECARD

Course Location:

Date:

Player	1	2	3	4	5	6	7	8	9
Par									

Player	10	11	12	13	14	15	16	17	18	Total
Par										

Notes:

MINIATURE GOLF SCORECARD

| Course Location: |
| Date: |

Player	1	2	3	4	5	6	7	8	9
Par									

Player	10	11	12	13	14	15	16	17	18	Total
Par										

Notes:

MINIATURE GOLF SCORECARD

Course Location:

Date:

Player	1	2	3	4	5	6	7	8	9
Par									

Player	10	11	12	13	14	15	16	17	18	Total
Par										

Notes:

MINIATURE GOLF SCORECARD

Course Location:

Date:

Player	1	2	3	4	5	6	7	8	9
Par									

Player	10	11	12	13	14	15	16	17	18	Total
Par										

Notes:

MINIATURE GOLF SCORECARD

| Course Location: |
| Date: |

Player	1	2	3	4	5	6	7	8	9
Par									

Player	10	11	12	13	14	15	16	17	18	Total
Par										

Notes:

MINIATURE GOLF SCORECARD

Course/Location:

Date:

Player	1	2	3	4	5	6	7	8	9
Par									

Player	10	11	12	13	14	15	16	17	18	Total
Par										

Notes:

MINIATURE GOLF SCORECARD

Course Location:

Date:

Player	1	2	3	4	5	6	7	8	9
Par									

Player	10	11	12	13	14	15	16	17	18	Total
Par										

Notes:

MINIATURE GOLF SCORECARD

| Course/Location: |
| Date: |

Player	1	2	3	4	5	6	7	8	9
Par									

Player	10	11	12	13	14	15	16	17	18	Total
Par										

Notes:

MINIATURE GOLF SCORECARD

Course Location:

Date:

Player	1	2	3	4	5	6	7	8	9
Par									

Player	10	11	12	13	14	15	16	17	18	Total
Par										

Notes:

MINIATURE GOLF SCORECARD

Course/Location:

Date:

Player	1	2	3	4	5	6	7	8	9
Par									

Player	10	11	12	13	14	15	16	17	18	Total
Par										

Notes:

MINIATURE GOLF SCORECARD

Course Location:

Date:

Player	1	2	3	4	5	6	7	8	9
Par									

Player	10	11	12	13	14	15	16	17	18	Total
Par										

Notes:

MINIATURE GOLF SCORECARD

Course/Location:

Date:

Player	1	2	3	4	5	6	7	8	9
Par									

Player	10	11	12	13	14	15	16	17	18	Total
Par										

Notes:

MINIATURE GOLF SCORECARD

Course Location:

Date:

Player	1	2	3	4	5	6	7	8	9
Par									

Player	10	11	12	13	14	15	16	17	18	Total
Par										

Notes:

MINIATURE GOLF SCORECARD

Course Location:

Date:

Player	1	2	3	4	5	6	7	8	9
Par									

Player	10	11	12	13	14	15	16	17	18	Total
Par										

Notes:

MINIATURE GOLF SCORECARD

Course Location:

Date:

Player	1	2	3	4	5	6	7	8	9
Par									

Player	10	11	12	13	14	15	16	17	18	Total
Par										

Notes:

MINIATURE GOLF SCORECARD

Course Location:
Date:

Player	1	2	3	4	5	6	7	8	9
Par									

Player	10	11	12	13	14	15	16	17	18	Total
Par										

Notes:

MINIATURE GOLF SCORECARD

Course Location:

Date:

Player	1	2	3	4	5	6	7	8	9
Par									

Player	10	11	12	13	14	15	16	17	18	Total
Par										

Notes:

MINIATURE GOLF SCORECARD

Course/Location:

Date:

Player	1	2	3	4	5	6	7	8	9
Par									

Player	10	11	12	13	14	15	16	17	18	Total
Par										

Notes:

MINIATURE GOLF SCORECARD

Course Location:

Date:

Player	1	2	3	4	5	6	7	8	9
Par									

Player	10	11	12	13	14	15	16	17	18	Total
Par										

Notes:

MINIATURE GOLF SCORECARD

Course Location:

Date:

Player	1	2	3	4	5	6	7	8	9
Par									

Player	10	11	12	13	14	15	16	17	18	Total
Par										

Notes:

MINIATURE GOLF SCORECARD

Course Location:

Date:

Player	1	2	3	4	5	6	7	8	9
Par									

Player	10	11	12	13	14	15	16	17	18	Total
Par										

Notes:

MINIATURE GOLF SCORECARD

Course/Location:
Date:

Player	1	2	3	4	5	6	7	8	9
Par									

Player	10	11	12	13	14	15	16	17	18	Total
Par										

Notes: